250

TIPS

FOR MAKING

LIFE WITH

ARTHRITIS

EASIER

OUR MISSION

The mission of the Arthritis Foundation is to support research to find the cure for and prevention of arthritis and to improve the quality of life for those affected by arthritis.

250

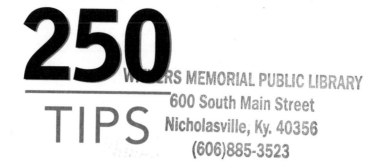

TIPS

FOR MAKING

LIFE WITH

ARTHRITIS

EASIER

Written by
SHELLEY PETERMAN SCHWARZ

for
THE ARTHRITIS FOUNDATION

LONGSTREET PRESS, INC.
Atlanta, Georgia

Published by Longstreet Press, Inc.
A subsidiary of Cox Newspapers,
A subsidiary of Cox Enterprises, Inc.
2140 Newmarket Parkway
Suite 122
Marietta, GA 30067

Printed in the United States of America

1st printing 1997

Library of Congress Catalog Card Number: 96-79812

ISBN 1-56352-381-7

CONTENTS

FOREWORD

As the title states, this book is designed to make your life with arthritis easier. But to get the most out of *250 Tips*, we suggest you do more than just read — you need to become an active partner in your own health care. That means finding out what type of arthritis you have and what management program is best for you. With your physician, you can determine what type of treatment you need and the best ways to cope with your illness — in other words, what to do, how to do it and, most important of all, what you can do to help yourself. Once you know more about the way your arthritis affects you, you can use the ideas in this book to help manage it.

Remember, you are the most important member of your health-care team. To ensure that you receive the best possible care for your arthritis, you should seek out individuals with experience in treating your particular condition. Your physician is important in making the diagnosis and determining the management approach that is right for you. You may need to see a rheumatologist, a physician who specializes in arthritic diseases. Other important members of your health-care team may include orthopaedic surgeons and other physicians, nurses, physiatrists, physical therapists, occupational therapists, social workers, pharmacists, dietitians, podiatrists and psychologists. The Arthritis Foundation chapter that serves your area can supply you with a list of local doctors who specialize in arthritis. Contacting the nearest university medical center may also help you find these individuals.

What is most important is that you work out a plan for your life with arthritis and find a role in which you feel comfortable. Your area Arthritis Foundation chapter has a number of programs and resources available to assist you in this endeavor.

After reading this book, you may find that not all of these tips are applicable to you. Many of them were designed for people who have a number of joints affected by arthritis and who experience associated fatigue. If you have questions about any of the *250 Tips*, consult your doctor or other members of your health-care team. Together, you can make decisions about your health that are right for you.

Doyt L. Conn, M.D.
Senior Vice President for Medical Affairs, Arthritis Foundation

Everyone, myself included, looks for ways to make life easier. Whether we're spring cleaning, preparing dinner or planting flowers, our goal is to save time and energy. When a chronic illness like arthritis enters the picture, life gets more complicated. Completing even simple tasks can become a challenge. Often we're forced to find new ways to accomplish the things we want to get done.

In my case, a 1979 diagnosis of multiple sclerosis (MS), and the years of increasing disability that followed, motivated me to simplify my life by organizing, streamlining and consolidating everyday tasks.

I learned to alternate periods of activity with periods of rest, to plan ahead and to take advantage of labor-saving devices and new technology. All these things conserve my energy, allowing me to do more of the things I want to do. Being organized and working smarter has also kept me more independent than I otherwise would have been.

In consulting with people at the Arthritis Foundation, I learned that many of the same principles apply to people with arthritis. This book offers tips and techniques for getting things done around the house while conserving energy and reducing wear and tear on your body. If you're willing to be flexible and creative, you'll be amazed by what you can do!

You'll learn dozens of ways to become better organized so you won't waste valuable energy searching for the things you need. You'll find ways to accomplish tasks quickly and efficiently. You'll discover low-cost community services and resources which you may not have known existed. In addition, you'll learn about easy-to-install devices designed to make your home and household activities more accessible.

Many of the products and devices I mention in the book are readily available in discount or hardware stores. To locate the more specialized items, I have three suggestions: 1) Contact an independent-living center in your area. Every state has several. Most centers have adaptive gadgets and devices you can borrow at no cost for a trial period. They also may have a vast computer database of the companies and manufacturers who make these products. The National Council on Independent Living (703/525-3406) may be able to assist you in finding the center nearest you. 2) Call local medical-supply companies and home-health and/or hospital-supply stores to see if they have the devices in stock. 3) Contact a hospital rehabilitation department and speak with an occupational or physical therapist about the product you're looking for. Whenever possible, try the device before purchasing it.

When you live with a chronic illness, it can be hard to predict good days and bad, let alone the future. I hope these tips help you increase the number of good days you have and encourage you to develop your own techniques for making life easier. I am convinced that finding ways to adapt, modify and simplify your life will give you the greatest opportunity to enjoy each day to the fullest.

Shelley Peterman Schwarz
Madison, Wisconsin
Syndicated columnist, author and professional speaker

ACKNOWLEDGMENTS

The Arthritis Foundation is proud to present *250 Tips for Making Life with Arthritis Easier.* The author is Shelley Peterman Schwarz, a woman who knows firsthand the value of creating shortcuts to make life easier. Lessons learned from dealing with her own chronic illness helped her to fill this book with clever and creative tips that are useful to anyone who's affected by any form of arthritis.

The tips listed in this book were carefully chosen and compiled by the author. Additional information was adapted from the popular *Guide to Independent Living for People with Arthritis,* published by the Arthritis Foundation in 1988. A panel of volunteer reviewers — including people with arthritis, physicians, occupational therapists and physical therapists — then carefully reviewed all of them to ensure that the information provided in this book is as helpful as possible.

Special thanks to Kathleen M. Haralson, P.T., M.L.A., Washington University Medical Center, St. Louis, Missouri; Pamela B. Harrell, O.T.R., C.H.T., Arthritis Care Center, Nashville, Tennessee; Julia McClanahan, Arthritis Foundation volunteer, Oak Ridge, Tennessee; Steve Miller, M.D., Emory Clinic Division of Rheumatology, Atlanta, Georgia; Bernard Rubin, D.O., University of North Texas Health Science Center, Fort Worth, Texas; and Linda Wilson, Arthritis Foundation volunteer, Andover, Massachusetts.

Thanks also to the following Arthritis Foundation reviewers: Janet Austin, Ph.D., vice president of American Juvenile

Arthritis Organization (AJAO) and Special Groups; Michele Boutaugh, B.S.N., M.P.H., vice president of Patient and Community Services; Doyt L. Conn, M.D., senior vice president of Medical Affairs; Leigh DeLozier, director of Consumer Publications; Cindy McDaniel, vice president of Publications; and Susan Percy, managing editor of *Arthritis Today*.

And, special thanks to Chuck Perry, Shannon Maggio, Jeannie Tarkenton, Amy Burton, Jill Dible and others at Longstreet Press for their help with this project.

If you have any questions as you read this book, write them down and take them with you to your doctor or therapist, or call your local office of the Arthritis Foundation.

Author: **Shelley Peterman Schwarz**
Editorial Director: **Adrienne Greer**
Art Director: **Jennifer Rogers**

INTRODUCTION

Whether you learned only recently that you have arthritis or have had it for a long time, you know that true independence is helping yourself. If you've discovered anything at all about living with arthritis, you've discovered that you may not need to change what you do, but perhaps how you do it. In these pages, you'll discover new uses for items you already have around the house. You'll learn new time- and energy-saving ways of doing daily tasks. You'll find out about unusual services and resources and how to access them. And you'll learn about unique products that make life easier, safer and less frustrating.

While this book is chock-full of practical advice, don't forget that all the members of your health-care team are valuable resources for information and advice. You may need to discuss some of the tips in this book with some of them before trying any of the suggestions. Together you can find the solution that will best suit your needs and lifestyle.

YOUR UNIQUE NEEDS

250 Tips for Making Life with Arthritis Easier is meant to be helpful to people with different types of arthritis and varying degrees and types of limitations. Because of the wide range of needs the book covers, some of its advice may not apply to you. In fact, some of these tips are geared toward people with severe arthritis, while other tips apply more to those with minor limitations. But differences aside, couldn't we all benefit from tips that make our lives easier?

Arthritis is not a single disease. There are more than 100 different types of arthritis, and each disease affects people in a different way. The word *arthritis* literally means *joint inflammation* (*arth* means *joint*, *itis* means *inflammation*). Problems associated with joints are the defining characteristic of most forms of arthritis, yet some arthritis-related conditions such as fibromyalgia or osteoporosis do not directly affect the joints but instead affect the muscles or bones. The unique way in which your disease affects you will determine what tips might be most helpful to you. For example:

- A person with **rheumatoid arthritis** that affects the joints of the hands may find that using a rubber jar opener or placing a rubber band around the lid makes opening a jar easier. See Tip #49.
- Someone with **osteoarthritis** of the knees, hips or lower spine may find that picking things up from the floor is a difficult task. Purchasing a reacher from a hardware store or simply using a long-handled barbecue fork can make this task much easier. See Tip #37.
- A child with **juvenile arthritis** may have difficulty holding a pencil. Wrapping a rubber band several times around the pencil or purchasing a rubber gripper for the pencil can make writing much easier. See Tip #16.
- Someone with **fibromyalgia** who has severe muscle pain and lacks energy may benefit from the many time-saving tips listed in this book. See Tips #1 and #2.

UNDERSTANDING AND MANAGING
YOUR ARTHRITIS

These tips, or any ideas that help you manage your arthritis, are just one element of a full-scale treatment plan. Educating yourself about your disease is another important element. You need to know that once you have been diagnosed with arthritis, you may have it for the rest of your life. However, arthritis does not mean a hopeless, downhill course. While researchers search for cures to various forms of arthritis, all types of arthritis can be treated and helped with proper management. Some types can be completely controlled or even cured.

The goal of modern arthritis care is to suppress disease activity and allow you to live as normal a life as possible. Some types of arthritis have periods of **flare** (active disease) and **remission** (minimal or no disease activity). Although you feel better during remissions, this does not mean that the arthritis is cured, just that it is controlled. It is important to take proper care of yourself at all times, not just when the disease is active.

COMMON SYMPTOMS OF ARTHRITIS

The most common symptoms of arthritis are joint pain, swelling and limitation of movement. The affected area may also appear red and feel warm to the touch. These symptoms are the result of a process called **inflammation,** which often affects the joints, or of cartilage deterioration.

Other signs of joint inflammation may include fatigue and stiffness, as well as involvement in other organs such as the skin (rashes), peripheral nerves (extremity pain and weakness) and salivary glands (mouth or eye dryness).

While treatment is most successful when started at an early stage of the disease, you and your physician can find ways to manage arthritis at any stage. Consult your physician for a treatment plan that's geared toward your symptoms. A combination of the following elements can make up an effective arthritis management program:

- **Medication**
- **Proper rest**
- **Joint protection**
- **Heat/cold application**
- **Specific exercises**
- **Energy conservation**
- **Adaptive equipment/splints**
- **Relaxation/stress management**
- **Surgery**

PROTECTING YOUR JOINTS

Joint protection, mentioned in the list above, involves a series of principles designed to help you reduce the stress on joints affected by arthritis. This means paying attention to how you use your body. Some postures and motions that are safe for most people may be harmful to you. Protecting your

joints will help reduce pain and inflammation, preserve your joints and help you stay as active as possible. Overuse and abuse of joints affected by arthritis can lead to:
- **Increased pain and swelling**
- **Further joint damage**
- **Loss of function**
- **Loss of independence**

Joint protection should be practiced all the times, not just on days when you have more pain. Here are some joint-protection principles to keep in mind:
- **Respect pain.**
  Pain is one of the body's signals that something is wrong. Although you may experience pain every day from your arthritis, harmful stress placed on your joints may cause even greater pain. That pain may last more than an hour or two following an activity or seem worse the next morning. This is a sign you have done more than you should. Try doing the task differently or getting help the next time. Help can come from another person or from one of the tips mentioned in this book designed to reduce joint stress.
- **Avoid improper postures or positions.**
  Posture refers to how your joints line up in relation to each other. Using the correct sitting position, with your head and back straight, neck supported and feet firmly planted on the floor, lets you sit comfortably and relaxed. A straight posture lying on your back, with one pillow under your head, is the best resting position for your joints.

- **Avoid staying in one position for a long time.**
  Keeping your joints in the same position can increase pain and stiffness. When writing a letter, for example, it is a good idea to relax and stretch your hand and arm every five minutes or so. Or, when watching television, get up and walk around every 20 to 30 minutes or so to avoid stiffness in your knees, hips and neck.
- **Use the strongest and largest joints and muscles for the job.**
  Avoid direct pressure on the small joints of your hands. Getting up from a chair can place a great deal of strain on your hands if you push yourself up with your fingertips. Instead of using your fingers or knuckles, use your palms to help you out of a chair. Or, sit in a chair that is higher than normal.
- **Avoid sustained joint activities.**
  Activities should be stopped or curtailed if they become too stressful for the joints. Rather than take a long walk without rest, you should make sure ahead of time that there will be benches to sit on along the way in case you need to rest. Or, rather than carry a package a long distance without resting, use a shopping cart from the start and push your load.
- **Maintain muscle strength and joint range of motion.**
  Preserving muscle strength and range of motion in the joints is important for maintaining the efficiency of your joints. Arthritis often reduces joint mobility and strength because of inflammation and pain. Gentle range-of-motion exercises

prescribed by your therapist can keep you mobile, and strengthening exercises will make sure the muscles around your joints can support the joint, relieving the stress. Aerobic-type exercises, too, are beneficial because they strengthen your heart. Always consult a health-care professional before beginning a new exercise regimen.

Community exercise programs designed to be gentle enough for people with arthritis or for older people are often available. Many of these programs are designed to work on flexibility and conditioning, and to provide social interaction. Consult the Arthritis Foundation chapter that serves your area for a list of programs available near you.

- **Use assistive devices and splints.**
  One way to protect your joints is to use labor-saving devices. Many different devices have been developed to make accomplishing tasks easier and more efficient. Many of the tips in this book suggest using assistive devices. Information about where to get them is included as well.

Some of the assistive devices mentioned in this book include:
  - **Wheeled laundry baskets (See Tip #59)**
  - **Enlarged key holders (See Tip #127)**
  - **Reachers (See Tip #37)**

Sometimes a splint or orthosis may be prescribed by your doctor or therapist. Or you may wonder if such devices would be helpful. A splint is a device designed to hold a limb or joint in a specific position to protect it. An orthosis is a brace usually made of stiff or hard material that restricts or increases motion of a body part. When used correctly, these devices can help rest or protect a joint, keep a joint in good alignment, stabilize a weak joint, prevent or correct joint damage, and reduce pain and inflammation. Consult your therapist or physician for more information on splints and orthoses.

Joint-Protection Principles
1. Respect pain.
2. Avoid improper postures or positions.
3. Avoid staying in one position for a long time.
4. Use the strongest and largest joints and muscles fo the job.
5. Avoid sustained joint activities.
6. Maintain muscle strength, joint range of motion and conditioning.
7. Use assistive devices and/or splints.

CONSERVING YOUR ENERGY

With many forms of arthritis, fatigue and energy loss are as much a problem as joint pain. Fatigue is often a hidden characteristic of arthritis. Though you look well to friends and family, you may, in fact, be low on energy and have to use more effort than other people to perform the same task.

Energy conservation is an important principle of arthritis management, teaching you to use energy wisely. Wearing yourself out will make your arthritis worse, not better. *250 Tips for Making Life with Arthritis Easier* suggests dozens of ways to do things that will save your energy and reduce fatigue. The following are ground rules that will help you feel better:

- **Balance activity with rest.**

  Pace yourself so that you are able to balance work periods with rest periods. Avoid doing two heavy chores in a row. With proper pacing, you will accomplish more than if you were to push yourself to get done sooner without a break.

- **Plan ahead.**

  Simplify your life as much as possible by planning and organizing your tasks wisely. This will help you space out your chores so you can rest in between. Combine activities that can be done at the same time to avoid spending extra energy. Always look for shortcuts and ways to combine steps.

- **Do what is most important first.**

  List and rank activities according to their importance. Do what is most important first. You may find some tasks that can be cut out or given to someone else.

- **Use principles of joint protection.**

  Simplify your work as much as possible. Use wheels, levers, lightweight objects and tools, and assistive devices to your advantage. Sit to work whenever possible. Overstressing yourself and your joints can add to your fatigue.

- **Get help from others.**
  Family and friends can share tasks and help plan your schedule. Your doctor and health-care team members can provide advice and new ideas and help you solve any problems you encounter.

Energy-Conservation Principles
1. Balance activity with rest.
2. Plan ahead.
3. Do what is most important first.
4. Use principles of joint protection.
5. Get help from others.

COPING WITH CHANGE

Dealing with a chronic disease like arthritis can cause psychological as well as physical problems. This is normal. Anger, sadness, frustration and fear are some of the many feelings people experience when they learn they have arthritis. Coping with changes in your body and in your ability to complete normal activities can be very stressful, and it can sometimes lead to depression. Counselors — including social workers and psychologists — may be able to provide support and help you cope with these changes. Your doctor may recommend that you see a counselor, and he or she can recommend names of counselors who may be helpful to you. Your local Arthritis Foundation chapter has support groups, educational programs and other resources to assist you in coping with these changes.

SUMMARY

Remember: The ultimate goal of *250 Tips* is exactly what the name states — to provide ways to make your life with arthritis easier, while reducing your pain and maximizing your independence. When you set goals for yourself, be realistic, be positive. Many challenges in life are successfully met with a positive attitude and a sense of humor. Actively managing your arthritis, while following the helpful tips included in this book, will make your life with arthritis the best it can be.

The Editors

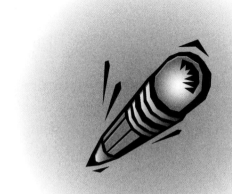

CHAPTER ONE

HOUSEHOLD BUSINESS

Paying bills, washing clothes, remembering to send a gift or greeting card — the business of managing your daily household activities requires energy and organization. Planning your home for convenience helps reduce the work to maintain it. Because stiffness, pain and fatigue usually accompany arthritis, becoming organized may fall to the bottom of your priorities. Don't let it. Organization can be the best gift you give yourself.

In this chapter, you'll learn ways to use your time more efficiently and manage your household paperwork. You'll also discover resources and services that will make these activities easier. Remember — you determine which ideas are appropriate for your household. By taking time to organize, you'll save your energy for when you really need it.

PLANNING AND USING YOUR TIME WISELY

1 Keep a "to do" list at the ready for those times when you feel ambitious. For those times when you can't seem to get anything done, keep an "all done" list, citing every task you complete, no matter how small. It feels good to realize how much you accomplish each day.

2 If you find it difficult to get everything done, try prioritizing your chores into categories like "must be done," "should be done" and "nice to get done." Begin the day by tackling the "must be done" items and take short breaks between them if necessary. Less important tasks and jobs can be assigned to family members or moved to another day.

CREATING HELPFUL "TO DO" LISTS

3 Small spiral-bound notebooks are great for jotting down information you need to remember and things you need to get done. If possible, you can carry the notebook with you to save steps retrieving it. Try keeping the notebook wherever you spend most of your busy hours, especially if you use a mobility aid like a walker or crutch. Attach one end of a piece of string or ribbon to a pen or pencil and the other end to the spiral binding, so you'll always have the notebook and a writing utensil handy.

If you use a wheelchair, it may be easier for you to use a calendar or notepad that goes where you go. You can wear an apron with pockets or tie the notepad to the side of your wheelchair. Keep the calendar or notepad and a pencil at hand, and you'll have your "to do" list with you wherever you go. Shorten or pleat the apron so the pockets are easy to reach into.

4 Large chalkboards or dry-erase boards are a good way to keep track of appointments and tasks if writing in small spaces is difficult. They are also nice because they eliminate your worries over losing papers and make entries easy to erase or update. Use different color markers or chalk to code messages for each family member. Check with your local office-supply store for styles and prices.

5 Electronic appointment calendars are helpful when writing is difficult. Shop your local electronics or office-supply store for one that is lightweight, with buttons that are easy to reach and push. If you have trouble finding one that you can use, try again in a few months. Because of new technology, the devices are rapidly evolving.

6 Self-sticking notes are great for helping you remember things that are to be done soon. Attach them to the door so you remember to take necessary items with you when leaving home. Or attach them to the bathroom mirror when you brush your teeth before bed so you are reminded of important appointments first thing when you get up in the morning.

ORGANIZING YOUR HOUSEHOLD PAPERWORK

7 If you have trouble turning the pages in a book or magazine, use a rubber finger or a tacky solution on your finger, or use the eraser end of a pencil to turn pages. Tacky solutions and rubber fingers can be found wherever office supplies are sold.

8 People who require frequent medical care may find it helpful to prepare a chronological list of medical treatments, surgeries, hospitalizations and medications taken. Take the list with you to your appointments so you only have to jot entries once. The list comes in handy, too, when answering physicians' and pharmacists' questions.

9 Shopping by mail is a great way to save time and energy. From prescriptions to clothing, you can purchase almost anything through the mail. When placing a mail order, write all the company's information in the memo area of your personal check. Then your canceled check will be a complete record of the purchase, should you need to contact the company for any reason.

10 Keep frequently used phone numbers handy to avoid having to lift a heavy telephone book when you need to look them up. Also, have the number for the poison control center and other emergency numbers by each telephone. If your phone has speed-dial options, you may want to program the numbers of those you call frequently. Or, you can use either a typed list of numbers or a Rolodex near each telephone.

If you use a list and are able to type, type the phone numbers for individuals you call frequently on one page. On a second page, type the numbers of frequently called businesses, doctors, etc. Photocopy both lists, staple them back to back and slip them into clear acetate sheets. Put one list near each phone in your house. If you use a Rolodex-type file, the cards can be updated easily and can be used for other information, such as clothing sizes, birthdays and anniversaries of persons in your file.

11. Keep your address and phone number affixed to each telephone in your home. If a visitor needs to summon help, he or she will have the necessary information.

12. At the beginning of the year, create a calendar for sending greeting cards. Begin with a new calendar that has a square for each day, and write the names of people celebrating birthdays, holidays, graduations, wedding anniversaries, etc., in the appropriate square. Then when you get to the store, purchase as many cards as you can. Sort the cards according to the month in which they must be mailed. File in an accordion file, or store in large envelopes. When those special days come up, simply pull out the card and send it. You might keep an extra envelope or file slot for sympathy, get well, new

baby and "just because" cards. The system is easy and prevents you from missing special dates when a flare keeps you at home.

13 If you have a home computer, use it to keep paperwork organized and to help family members who must assist with your personal business. Create a document entitled WHEREIT.IS in which you list the location of important or valuable papers. For security purposes, protect the document with a password which you have given only to those who might need to access the file. Keep a backup of the file on a floppy disk in a separate location, like in a safe-deposit box or at the home of a family member.

If you don't have a computer, write or type a master list and keep it in a safe location away from home, such as in a safe-deposit box.

WRITING MADE EASIER

14 Reduce the writing you must do by using a computerized or stamped image of your signature. You can create a computerized image of your signature at print shops that have computer scanners. Load the scanned image onto your home computer to electronically sign correspondence.

If you don't have a computer, you can purchase a signature stamp from your financial institution or office-supply store. Check with your bank to see if the signature stamp can be used on your checks as well as other documents.

15. If you have a lot of writing to do, try using roller-ball pens. They glide more easily on paper than felt-tip pens or pencils or even ball points.

16. If holding a pen or pencil is difficult, try using a rubber grip. Make your own by having someone twist a rubber band around your pen or pencil several times. Push the rubber band into position just below the spot where your fingers rest. If you need a more substantial grip, purchase a small, triangular rubber grip from a school- or office-supply store. The grips have a hole in the center and you simply push them into position on your pens or pencils. Large-grip or comfort-grip pens are also available and make writing easier.

17. If writing checks is difficult due to vision or fine motor control problems, there are a variety of ways to make the work easier. You can make a check template by asking someone to cut spaces out of thin cardboard or other material to match the lines on your checks. To use, place the template on top of the check and use the openings as guides for writing.

As an alternative, you can order embossed or large-size checks from your check printer. The raised lines on both kinds of checks serve as writing guides for completing the checks.

18   Reduce the amount of writing you must do when paying bills, sending cards or completing forms. Purchase either a self-inking return-address stamp or preprinted, self-stick labels. Stamps and labels can be ordered in a variety of font styles from office-supply stores, print shops or wherever stationery is sold. Use them to affix your return address on envelopes and to fill out the name/address sections of documents you must complete.

SPECIAL ENERGY-SAVING TECHNIQUES

19   Make gift shopping easier by taking with you a list of the sizes and measurements of people for whom you need to buy gifts. Include addresses for those who live out of town and ask the store to wrap and mail the gifts directly to the recipients. By doing this, you don't have to carry heavy packages which may strain your hand and elbow joints, or make extra exhausting trips to the post office.

20   If you prefer wrapping your holiday gifts yourself, do so as soon as you purchase them so you won't have to fuss with them as the holidays become more hectic. When wrapping lots of gifts at one time, use an adjustable ironing board as a table. You can reduce strain on your neck and back while you work by raising or lowering the height of the ironing board to suit your needs. As an alternative to wrapping gifts, purchase some of the brightly colored gift bags which are widely available.

21 Save steps when you need to get the attention of someone in the basement. Instead of tackling a flight of dark, steep stairs, switch the lights on and off from the top of the stairs.

22 Getting plenty of rest is key in managing arthritis. Consider having your answering machine take your phone calls when you need to rest or when you want to complete a task without interruption.

23 If limited hand strength makes scissors difficult to use, try using a seam ripper to clip coupons and newspaper articles. See also Tip #84.

24 Use a large 24- to 30-point typeface when creating or reading a document on the computer. It's easier on your eyes and helps you catch more mistakes.

HELPFUL RESOURCES AND SERVICES

25 If it's difficult for you to retrieve your mail from a distant mailbox, you may qualify to have your mail delivered directly to your door. Known as "hardship delivery," this service is available by submitting a written request with appropriate medical documentation to your local postmaster. Call the post office near you for information. If your request is denied and you want to appeal the decision, contact the Consumer Advocate, U.S. Postal Service, 475 L'Enfant Plaza, Washington, DC 20260-6320, or call the national customer referral line at 202/268-2284.

26 If using a telephone directory is difficult, you may be able to receive directory-assistance services free of charge. Your doctor will need to document exactly how your arthritis prevents you from using a telephone book to obtain addresses and phone numbers. Call your telephone company to see if the service is available in your area.

27 If you don't have an intercom system in your home, you may be able to use your telephones to signal and speak to family members in other rooms of the house. Many telephone companies offer the "revertive calling" feature in their service that allows you to use your telephone as an intercom. Simply dial your telephone number, wait for a busy signal and hang up the receiver. All the phones in your house will ring. Individuals in different rooms can pick up the handsets and speak to each other without hearing a dial tone in the background. If you don't currently have this feature, contact your local telephone company and find out when it will be available.

28 If getting out of the house to vote is a problem, consider contacting the city clerk in your area for a permanent absentee ballot. You will receive a ballot before each election so you can cast your vote by mail.

29 Do your banking from home if getting to the bank is difficult. Ask the bank for stamped, self-addressed envelopes for mailing deposits and payments. The bank will process your transactions and return the receipts to you. If possible, arrange for your checks to be automatically deposited to your account.

30 Most banks offer a bank-by-phone service that allows you to dial a local or toll-free number to check your account balance, the amount of your last deposit, and previous checks that have cleared. Some banks even allow you to apply for a loan or conduct transactions such as account transfers by phone. Ask your bank's customer service representative if this service is available.

31 Some banks will send a representative to your home to help you with your bill paying and record keeping. Shop around and choose a bank that offers the services you need. Or ask your bank to pay your household bills electronically. Each month, utility payments (and some others) will automatically be paid, and you'll receive documentation of the transactions.

32 For a nominal charge, the U.S. Postal Service offers stamped envelopes that include your preprinted return-address label. All you have to do is stuff and seal the envelopes, which are available in lots of 50. To place an order, call 800/STAMP-24. For those times when you have to stamp envelopes yourself, purchase large commemorative or self-adhesive stamps and oversized return-address labels.

33 Call your local post office and ask for a Stamps by Mail brochure. Your letter carrier will bring the brochure to you with your next mail delivery and you'll be able to order stamps, postcards, envelopes, etc., by mail at no extra charge. Just send the completed form and your payment to the main post office (the address is on the form). Within a day or two, your letter carrier will deliver your order with your mail. You don't even have to pay postage or delivery charges on your order.

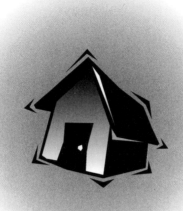

CHAPTER TWO

HOUSEHOLD
ORGANIZATION

If you have arthritis, you will do better if you give more fore-thought and planning to all tasks — even simple ones. When your joints are inflamed or painful, you may not feel like going upstairs to get something you forgot. Simply reaching up for an item on a closet shelf can be difficult when joints are stiff. Before you experience a flare, you need to take certain precautions as you do all your daily activities. This chapter will help you organize your household so that items are easier to find, store, retrieve and maintain. Even if you feel that some of these tips may not apply to you, becoming organized in advance of a painful flare can reduce stress to your joints and help conserve energy.

ARRANGING CLOSETS AND DRAWERS

34 Cardboard boxes with dividers, like those in which liquor bottles are shipped, make great closet organizers; each cubicle can store a pair of shoes. Cover the box with self-adhesive paper for a more finished look.

35 Keep a laundry basket in every bedroom closet. The baskets are handy for holding and transporting laundry to the laundry room. Make it a household rule that each member of the family be responsible for transporting his basket to and from the laundry room. If lifting a laundry basket is a problem, purchase a laundry cart or hamper on wheels. Check your local housewares or discount department store for styles, sizes and prices.

36 Create a lower bar in a closet by suspending two equal lengths of rope from either end of the existing closet bar. (The length of ropes will depend on how low you want the new bar to hang.) Attach another bar to the ends of the ropes. You'll double the hanging space for short items like blouses, shirts and skirts. If reaching up for something is a problem, keep frequently used items on the lower bar.

37 Keep a reacher inside your closet to pick up items from the floor or to aid in reaching hanging items. Reachers extend your reach up to 36 inches, and there are many styles to choose from. Some will pick up paper or small objects. Some are magnetic to help you retrieve metal objects. Some operate like scissors; others work like tongs. You can purchase reachers from home-health supply stores and catalogs. As an alternative, fireplace tongs, barbecue tongs and aquarium tongs also make great reachers. See also Tip #51.

38 Pulling to open stuck drawers can be hard on swollen fingers, wrists or elbows. To make drawers easier to open, spray the runners with a dry silicone spray. Adding drawer stops to drawers will prevent them from pulling out and falling to the floor. Both items are available at hardware or building-supply stores. You may also find it helpful to have someone tie loops onto your drawer pulls so that you can open the drawer with your arm instead of with sore fingers.

SIMPLIFYING STORAGE

39 Organize household items by storing like things together and keeping them near the place in which they will be used. For example, sports equipment might be stored in the garage, sewing supplies and notions in the sewing room closet, and herbs and spices in the drawer nearest the stove. See also Tip #153.

40 Store mittens, scarves and hats in a hanging shoe bag inside the coat closet.

41 Square plastic baby-wipe containers make perfect lightweight storage containers for small items like cards, crayons, hair accessories and first-aid supplies.

42 Shoe boxes are great for storing things like cookie cutters, craft supplies, appliance cords, hair ribbons and barrettes. Often, shoe stores have empty boxes they're willing to give you. You can paint the box or cover it with an adhesive-backed paper so it's more attractive, and leave it out on a shelf or countertop. If you store the boxes on a closet shelf, label the outside of each box for easy retrieval.

43 If you have arthritis in your hands, you know how difficult it can be to untangle necklaces. Instead of storing them in a jewelry box, try using a revolving tie rack for organizing your favorite necklaces.

44 Store tools on a pegboard and use a marking pen to outline the space for each tool. You can tell at a glance if a tool is missing.

45 Store out-of-season items, like clothing and holiday decorations, in sweater boxes that fit under the bed to save trips to the basement or attic storage areas. You can find plastic, metal or cardboard sweater boxes at discount department stores or wherever clothing organizers are sold.

USING HELPFUL HOUSEHOLD PRODUCTS

46 Wrap the handles of household and outdoor tools like brooms, shovels, rakes and mops with foam pipe insulation for easier gripping. The foam tubing is available in a variety of diameters. It's slit on one side so it's easy to install. For indoor tools, keep the tubing in place with rubber bands or duct tape. For outdoor tools, wrap the handles with brightly colored electrical tape so the tools are easier to find in the grass. You can find the tubing at most hardware or home-improvement stores.

47 Whenever possible, use long-handled cleaning devices to help reduce strain on your joints. You might try using a long-handled paint roller to apply floor wax or a long-handled mop to clean your bathtub without having to bend or work on your hands and knees. Long-handled dusters can help reduce excessive reaching. Wearing a splint can protect your joints from the extra strain caused by mopping and sweeping.

48 Dycem is a unique product that has many uses. It is a thin vinyl-like material with a tacky, rubbery feel. When placed under an object, the object won't move or slide. When you cut a strip of Dycem and fasten it with tape around a pen, drinking glass, razor, TV remote control, etc., the object will not slip out of your hands. Home-health stores or hospital rehabilitation centers can help you locate this product.

49 A rubber waffle-type gripper keeps jars from turning so you can open them with just one hand. Simply set a jar on top of the gripper and you can unscrew the lid without the bottle turning. You can also place the gripper over the lid to make unscrewing the lid easier. Find the grippers in the kitchen gadgets section of grocery and discount stores.

50 Use a partially filled hot-water bottle as a pad to kneel on when washing floors or working in the garden.

51 If it's difficult to reach above your shoulders or to grasp objects from a wheelchair, keep a reacher nearby. As an alternative, fireplace tongs, barbecue tongs and aquarium tongs also make great reachers. See also Tip #37.

52 Wearing rubber gloves makes it easier for weak hands to grasp objects and protects hands from cleaning chemicals. To make the gloves easier to put on and take off, sprinkle a little cornstarch or baby powder inside each one. If they're still difficult to remove, try holding your hands under cold water and then pulling them off. If one of the gloves gets a hole in it (usually the one for your dominant hand), keep the mate. The next time another dominant-hand glove wears out, turn the mate you saved inside out and you'll have a new pair of gloves.

53 Squeeze bottles can be used to dispense everything from moisturizing lotion and liquid soap to ketchup and salad dressing. There are no tops to unscrew or heavy bottles to lift. Reuse empty liquid soap or lotion bottles, or buy the bottles at discount or bathroom supply stores.

54 Use needle-nosed pliers or long-handled surgical tweezers if you need help grasping or picking up small objects like strands of thread, straight pins and pills.

55 If reading is difficult, try keeping several magnifying glasses in various locations around the house. Use one in the kitchen and one in the bathroom to help you read labels, ingredients panels and directions. Keep one with the telephone book. You might want to carry one with you to use at a grocery store or restaurant, or keep one in the car for reading maps.

56 Turntables, also known as Lazy Susans, make a variety of items easier to reach. Use them inside your refrigerator and kitchen and bathroom cabinets. Put one in the middle of the kitchen or dining room table to make it easier to reach napkins, condiments and other items. Turntables are available at most discount department stores.

MOVING THINGS FROM HERE TO THERE

57 If you have limited use of your hands, experiment with ways to carry items with you and keep your hands free. Try using a drill holster to hold a cordless phone or TV remote control. You can snap the holster to the leg of a wheelchair or to a scooter basket. You'll find drill holsters where power tools are sold.

58 You can also keep your hands free by wearing an apron that has pockets across the front. The pockets can hold anything you need handy or have to carry from one place to another — canned goods, cooking utensils, scissors, nails and a hammer, masking tape and so on. Alternatively, a fishing vest is another way to hold many small items. Such vests have a number of pockets and can be purchased at many sporting goods stores.

59 Moving items around the house is easier if you use a wheeled cart. Some that work well are tea and utility carts, collapsible luggage carriers and wheeled laundry carts.

If you load a tea or utility cart with dishes, glasses and silverware, you can set or clear the table in just one trip. Consider using a cart to move cleaning supplies or heavy items around the house. You might also use one to move groceries from the car to the house. Check your local discount department store for sizes, styles and prices.

60 If you use a wheelchair, try keeping a shallow corrugated box on your lap in which to place items that need to be carried from place to place.

61 Carrying items in a backpack or waistpack instead of in a shoulder-slung purse or bag will help you keep your balance while walking. It will also relieve stress on your shoulders and on the joints in your hands.

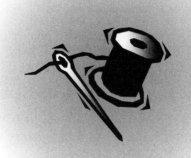

CHAPTER THREE

HOUSEHOLD
CHORES

Washing and waxing, cooking and cleaning — unless you have the luxury of a housekeeper or family member who can provide these services for you, the burden of maintaining your house may fall on you. The more extensive your arthritis, the more you should consider delegating some jobs to others. Hire someone to clean your gutters. Have your teenagers or neighborhood kids help you with cleaning the oven or sweeping the porch.

This chapter offers some tips to make your routine household chores, meal planning and grocery shopping easier. Remember, though, to listen to your body. Both work and leisure activities are important, but be careful not to overdo them. Pace yourself, take rest breaks and ask for help when you need it. Your family and friends will understand you better if you share your feelings with them and let them know how they can help you.

HOUSEKEEPING MADE EASIER

62 If you live in a multi-level house, save time and energy by keeping a set of cleaning supplies (brooms, cleansers, rubber gloves, etc.) on each level of the house. It's also a good idea to keep small cleaning supplies in a storage bin or bucket that has a handle. You can carry the bin with you as you work. Avoid carrying too heavy a load, however, because the handles can pull on painful finger joints.

63 Stop clutter before it accumulates. Picking up around the house daily accomplishes more than a monthly heavy cleaning and isn't as likely to exhaust you. Work in rhythm, playing music if it helps.

64 If you live in a multi-level house, keep a small basket near the stairs to hold items that need to be taken to rooms on a different floor. Collect the items throughout the day, and, to avoid carrying heavy loads, have someone carry the basket of items up or down the stairs for you and put the items in their proper places.

65 If a full container of dishwasher detergent is too difficult to lift and pour, have someone pour some of the detergent into a small, plastic pitcher. Each time you run the dishwasher, just pour what you need from the smaller container.

66 Polish chrome fixtures quickly and easily by wiping them with rubbing alcohol.

67 Dusting can be frustrating when hands are affected by arthritis. Save energy when dusting by using an old sock as a dust cloth. Simply dampen the sock with furniture polish and slip it over your hand. When dusting, work with your fingers as straight as possible, and use both hands, not just one. This way your arms and shoulders do most of the work.

68 If you do not have a dust mop, try dusting hardwood floors using tack cloth that has been wound around the end of a broom. Tack cloth removes dust quickly and can be purchased at your local hardware store.

69 Dust behind large appliances and other hard-to-reach areas using a yardstick or child's play broom. Cover one end of the yardstick with a sock and secure it with a rubber band. If using the broom, simply pin a dust rag around the bristle end.

70 Use a permanent marker or nail polish to mark quart, half-gallon and gallon lines on your cleaning bucket. The markings will make it easy to mix the right amount of cleaning solutions.

71 Select a vacuum that is as lightweight as possible but still has the power you require. Upright vacuum cleaners are easier to use than other models. They also allow you to walk as you vacuum, or even work from a chair. Standing still while pushing and pulling the vacuum puts more stress on your back.

72 Consider doing just light floor cleaning yourself and delegating the heavier work to other members of the family or to a housekeeper. For light sweeping, try using a child's play broom or a short-handled whisk broom so you can sit to sweep the floor. Both are lightweight and easy to control. Or, to avoid bending, use a carpet sweeper.

73 To save steps and recycle at the same time, use the plastic bags you receive from grocery and discount stores as liners in each wastebasket. Put several empty bags into the bottom of the wastebaskets and use one bag as the liner. When the liner bag is full, discard it and pull up another bag from the bottom of the wastebasket to use as the new liner.

IMPROVING HOME MAINTENANCE

74 To make cleaning the fireplace easier, spread a large piece of heavy-duty aluminum foil underneath the grate before you arrange the firewood and kindling. After the ashes from the fire cool, simply discard the foil. Or try lightly misting the cooled ashes with water to make them easier to remove.

75 A screwdriver magnetizer/demagnetizer helps you hold screws in place while working. To magnetize a screwdriver, simply pass the tool through the magnetizer's hole a few times. When you remove the screwdriver, it's magnetized and screws will cling to it. If you touch the screw to the tool, the magnetic field will hold it there. It's much easier than gripping a tiny screw and controlling the screwdriver at the same time. (If the magnetic pull isn't strong enough to hold a screw securely, leave the magnetizer on the screwdriver while you're using it.)

To demagnetize the screwdriver, just stroke the tool against the grooved channel on the outside of the magnetizer. Magnetizers can be purchased at local hardware or electronic stores. Be sure to keep this product away from your home computer and computer disks, or your data may be scrambled.

76 To sand a piece of furniture or other wooden object that has unusual corners or angles, wrap sandpaper around a small block of wood or something comparable, like a deck of playing cards. Secure with a rubber band.

DOING THE LAUNDRY

77 If a container of laundry detergent is too difficult to lift and pour, have someone pour some of the detergent into a small, plastic pitcher that's easier to handle.

78 Make your washer and dryer easier to use. If you have trouble bending to get clothes in and out of the dryer, have the dryer raised to a comfortable height (perhaps 6 to 8 inches higher) by setting it on top of a wooden platform. Keep a reacher nearby for moving clothes from the washer to the dryer or from the dryer to the laundry basket. The reacher will also come in handy if any clothes fall to the floor.

79 Use a sheet of fabric softener to clean the lint trap in your clothes dryer. The treated sheets attract the lint, making it easier to remove.

80 Here are two options to avoid setting up a full-size ironing board: Try buying a mini ironing board that you can place on a table top. Or, instead, consider purchasing a hand-held steamer which completely eliminates the need for an ironing board. Check for styles and prices at your local discount department store.

81 If you must iron on a full-size board, lower the board to a height that allows you to sit comfortably while ironing. Also, choose a chair that permits you to sit with correct posture.

SEWING AND OTHER HANDIWORK

82 When doing any type of needlework, always sit in good light in a chair with proper support. Poor posture increases fatigue as well as the likelihood of muscle spasms, stiffness and pain. Organize all your materials within easy reach and have your work at a comfortable height that keeps your arms relaxed.

83 When sewing, try using straight pins with large balls on top or glass-headed quilting pins. These are easier to grasp than standard straight pins. Also, to avoid bending to pick up pins that you drop while sewing, use a yardstick that has a magnet glued to the bottom or a magnetized screwdriver.

84 Sewing and larger mending jobs are easier if you use loop scissors or lightweight electric scissors rather than manual shears. Sit at a table to cut fabric and slide it toward you rather than bending over it. For smaller tasks, use a seam ripper. You can find these products at sewing shops or discount department stores.

85 Try a magnifying glass that hangs from your neck to magnify your sewing or craft project. These unique products can be found at sewing or craft stores.

86 Here are a few suggestions for threading needles: Try to thread a needle by sticking the needle into an apple or a potato and placing it on a shelf or counter that's at eye level. Or purchase self-threading needles from a fabric store. There is a small indentation near the eye of the needle where you rest the thread. Holding both sides of the thread, you give a quick pull, and the thread slips between a narrow opening in the needle and is automatically threaded. (There's also a second eye which you can use to thread the needle normally.) You can also have someone pre-thread needles with colors you use often so your needles are always ready to use.

87 Make hemming someone's slacks or skirt easier by using a plumber's plunger to mark the hem length. Simply mark the plunger handle at the desired length, then move the plunger across the floor and around the garment. Since the plunger stands by itself, it leaves your hands free to pin or mark the hem with chalk.

Hold the hem in place with iron-on hemming tape. Or, use spring-type clothespins or hair clips; they're easier to handle than pins, they eliminate the need to baste the hem, and they don't put holes in the fabric.

88 When replacing a lost button, first tape it to the garment with cellophane tape. After you've made a few stitches to secure the button to the garment, remove the tape and finish sewing.

89 When sewing together knitted or crocheted projects, keep the two pieces together with the long, plastic hair picks used to hold brush rollers in place. The picks are easier to see and grasp than straight pins, and they keep the seams better in place.

SHOPPING FOR GROCERIES

90 After a flare, before you go out shopping, call stores in your area to find out how accessible they are. (You may not have thought of your usual stores in this way before.) Competitive prices and convenient location are important, but so is your comfort. Ask about aisle widths, lighting, parking, restrooms and motorized shopping carts.

91 Some grocery stores offer special services to help shoppers select and pick up the items they need. Smaller neighborhood stores may provide home delivery; you simply call in your order and, for a fee, they will deliver groceries to your home. Larger chain stores may not deliver, but they sometimes maintain a list of companies that offer pick up and delivery from their store. You may be able to request that the store assemble a few items that you need and have them ready for you to pick up at a specified time. Call stores in your area to ask about the services you would find most helpful.

92 Do your grocery shopping when the store is least busy. During those times you may be able to get special services not available during busier times of the day. For example, the person at the deli counter could dice your onions and place them in a plastic bag. Perhaps the cashier could break the seals of hard-to-open jars. Call the store to find out what days and times are least busy.

93 Before shopping, prioritize your grocery list, marking important items. If you run out of energy at the store, you'll be sure to get the items you most need. You might write your list on the back of an envelope. Then put your coupons inside. Clip the envelope to the grocery cart so your hands will be free to push the cart and retrieve your items.

94 Stock up on staples like paper products, boxed and canned goods and other frequently used items. This way, you can make sure you shop when you feel most energetic.

95 If you would like assistance in getting from the grocery store parking lot to the store, try calling ahead to have a store employee meet you at your car.

96 If you have children, take them with you to the grocery store and let them help you retrieve products from the shelves. Depending on their ages, you might say, "Find the box with white flowers on it," "the 12-ounce bottle of salad dressing," or "the spaghetti sauce with mushrooms and garlic." It takes a little more time, but it's a great learning experience for the kids and helps protect your joints from injury due to lifting and reaching.

97 Try wearing a glove with leather on the palm and fingers to help you grasp glass bottles and metal cans while grocery shopping. The glove will also keep your hands warm while handling cold foods.

98 If you have Raynaud's phenomenon (a condition in which poor blood flow results in pain and skin color changes in affected parts of the body), protect your hands from cold by wearing thick gloves or mittens to reach into the freezer at the grocery store and at home.

99 Ask the person bagging the groceries to pack frozen and refrigerated items separately from foods that don't require refrigeration, and to avoid packing bags too full. When you arrive home you can carry just the bags containing the cold items and put them directly into the refrigerator or freezer. The rest can be carried in later, after you've rested or when you have help available.

CARING FOR HOUSEPLANTS

100 To dust the leaves on indoor plants, wear a pair of cotton gloves (or old socks) and dampen them with warm water. With one hand on top and one on the bottom, use both hands to wipe off the leaves.

101 If watering houseplants is a problem because it's difficult to carry the watering can, consider purchasing an indoor plant hose from your local garden-supply center. The hose is lightweight and easy to manage. Attach it to the kitchen or bathroom sink. In most homes you'll be able to reach all the plants on one floor.

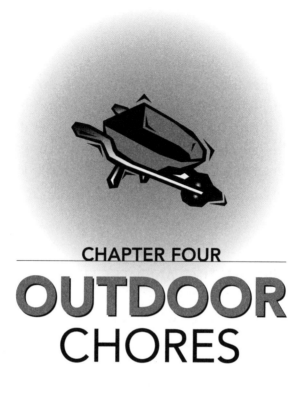

CHAPTER FOUR

OUTDOOR
CHORES

Having arthritis doesn't mean you must give up the activities and hobbies you enjoy or need to do, such as yard work or gardening. Keeping up your grounds, even if they are small, is an activity that can be beneficial if you don't overdo it, and if you use proper techniques to protect your hands, back, hips and legs.

You may have to be creative in coming up with new ways to plant flowers or water the lawn. Look for techniques that put less stress on your joints and conserve your energy. When working outside your house, you will need a method for moving items around. It is also important for you to carefully and realistically decide which jobs are worthwhile for you to do and which should be delegated.

Remember to use good posture and follow your joint-pro-tection principles to prevent injury or strain. Keeping the grounds of your home beautiful will be easier if you follow the tips in this chapter. Most items mentioned are available in the garden center of your local discount department or home-improve-ment store.

GARDENING TIPS AND TECHNIQUES

102 Planting seeds is easier when done standing up. One way to avoid bending while planting is to use a PVC pipe to guide seeds into the soil. Start with a 3-foot section of 1- or 2-inch-diameter pipe. Cut one end on the diagonal. Keeping the diagonally cut end of the pipe touching the ground, drop seeds down the pipe where you want the plants to grow. Cover the seeds by dropping soil down the pipe, or by care-fully scraping soil over the seeds with the end of the pipe. Or, for an easy alternative, fill a salt shaker or spice bottle that has a shaker top with seeds. After preparing the soil, simply shake the bottle over the areas you want to plant.

103 It's easier to plant seeds the appropriate distance apart if you use a seed-sowing board. To make your own, have someone drill evenly spaced holes in a Masonite board. Lay the board on the ground and drop the seeds through each hole.

104 Growing flower gardens is easy with pre-seeded, 12-foot "flower carpets." The seeds are embedded into a carpet of mulch so there are no individual seeds to handle. Just loosen the soil to a depth of 3 to 4 inches and rake smooth. Roll out the carpet, cut to size and remove the paper covering. Cover with $1/8$ inch of soil to guard against strong winds, and soak with a fine mist until saturated. Water once a day until plants are 3 to 4 inches tall. (Seedlings appear in about 1 to 2 weeks, flowers in 6 to 8 weeks.) The preseeded carpets are available at nurseries, greenhouses and mail-order companies.

105 Purchase plants from nurseries to eliminate the painstaking work of growing plants from seeds. Ask the salesperson to point out particularly hardy plants and those that require little care.

106 Pulling weeds is easier if the ground is moist. Do your work in the morning when the ground is still wet with dew or after a big rainfall, or lightly moisten the ground using a garden hose. You might consider purchasing a long-handled weeding tool from a nursery or garden shop. Ask for help in making your selection of weeding tools.

107 Sit on a garden stool or chair to work in the garden or flower bed, and use well-made child-size rakes or shovels to work the soil. Some of these specially designed garden seats have self-locking wheels and storage compartments.

108   Use a plastic sports-drink bottle with a flexible straw to water hard-to-reach plants. Squeeze the bottle and the water runs out of the container.

109   A trellis or container garden is a great way to grow your favorite vegetables without the work and strain of a regular garden. Begin by selecting a location like a low window ledge, balcony, walkway or patio that's easy to reach and near a water supply.

     Be sure to choose an appropriate container. Clay pots work well because they are porous and allow excess water and salt to escape. If you prefer, you can use the clay pots as liners inside more decorative pots, such as barrels, bushel baskets or window boxes. If the container is large, put it where you want it to stay before you fill it with dirt; after filling, it may be too heavy to move. Almost any plant can be grown in a container. Remember, though, that most container-grown plants need to be watered more often than plants grown in the ground.

110   If getting up and down makes growing a garden difficult, try cultivating a garden in a raised bed. Have a flower bed built out of lumber so that it is raised to about 34 inches or a height that is comfortable for you.

111   For easy care of outside hanging plants, hang them from a pulley rather than a hook. Attach a rope to the hanger on the plant, thread the rope through the pulley, and pull the plant up. Tie the rope "figure 8" style around two nails on the wall near the plant. You can simply unloop the "figure 8" and lower the plant for watering or pruning.

112 Use garden tools that have enlarged or padded handles to reduce stress on your hands from gripping.

113 Protect your hands while gardening by purchasing gardening gloves that are one or two sizes too large. Then stuff foam or sponge-type padding in and around your fingers. When handling thorny plants, try using a quilted oven mitt.

TAKING CARE OF YARDWORK, GARBAGE AND WINTER CHORES

114 When raking and removing leaves, try using clothespins to clip leaf bags to a fence. You'll be able to keep both hands free to fill the bags. If you don't have a fence, try filling a paper grocery bag with some of the leaves and lawn clippings. Insert the partially filled grocery bag into the larger bag so the lawn bag will prop open.

115 Mowing the grass is a task that can put excessive demands on your body. Starting a push mower with a pull chain can be harmful to your back and hard on your hands. What's more, pushing a mower can be stressful for the lower back and hips if they are not properly supported. You may want to leave this task to someone else. If you have to mow the grass, select a riding mower with controls that are easy to operate and a seat with full back support. Consult your local hardware or yard-equipment supplier for recommendations.

116 The effects of winter weather can be a problem if you live in a northern or elevated region. When snow is on the ground, try using a round metal or plastic disk-type sled to pull garbage bags to the curb. To make snow shoveling easier, apply an aerosol vegetable spray or furniture polish to the shovel. The snow will slide off easily.

117 Handling garbage is an almost daily task. You may want to consider purchasing a trash compactor to reduce the handling of everyday trash in your home. Then, find a light-weight, wheeled container to transport trash to the street, or ask someone else to take it out.

118 If you must move wood, save your back, hips and hands by using a carrier with wheels. If you have no carrier, follow these tips for carrying wood: Rather than grasping wood with your hands, carry loads of wood close to your body on your forearms to reduce stress on your back. Remember, it is better to carry several partial loads than one heavy load that causes you to strain.

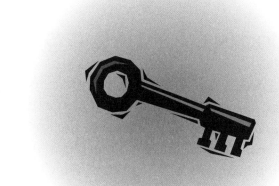

CHAPTER FIVE

THE ACCESSIBLE HOME

Making your home as comfortable as possible is a priority for everyone, especially if you have arthritis. There's no need for costly remodeling or structural changes to make your home more accessible. In this chapter, you'll learn tips as simple as making a doorknob easier to grasp and soundproofing your home for quieter rest periods. You'll also discover which businesses offer the materials or supplies to help you get these tasks done. As we've noted before, some of these tips may be particularly helpful for people with a certain type of arthritis. If you have questions, check with your physician to determine which ones are right for you.

USING DOORS, DOORWAYS, KEYS AND LOCKS

119 If turning a doorknob is difficult, have someone wind a few rubber bands around the largest part of the knob. The rubber bands increase the diameter of the knob and make it easier to grasp. To increase the diameter even more, cover knobs with padded doorknob covers, which are available at most hardware stores.

120 Make doors easier to open by installing lever handles. Hardware and building-supply stores have many styles to choose from.

121 If someone in your home uses a wheelchair, you can widen the doorways up to an inch and a half by installing offset hinges. The hinges allow the door to swing out and away from the doorway opening. They are easy to install using the existing holes and screws, and they require no cutting or drilling. You can find the hinges at many hardware or building-supply stores.

122 Here are two ways to make it easier to close doors behind you: 1) Tie a string or cord from the doorknob. Take hold of the cord as you begin to walk through the doorway, and the door will shut behind you as you walk. 2) Attach one cup hook in the door near the knob and another in the door jamb on the hinge side. Tie a string or chain from one hook to the other. As you go through the doorway, pull the string and the door will close behind you.

123 Doors that are too long and hard to open because they rub on the floor can be adjusted without removing them. Put a large piece of sandpaper on the floor under the door and move the door back and forth a few times. You may need to put some newspapers under the sandpaper so there will be a good contact with the bottom of the door. The sandpaper smooths the bottom of the door to prevent it from rubbing on the floor. As a result, the doors are easier to open and are easier on your joints.

124 To prop open heavy doors, use a tablespoon as a doorstop. Turn the spoon upside down and push the handle under the door.

125 To protect your doors from wheelchair scratches, put a clear Lucite, chrome or brass kick plate on the bottom of the door. You can purchase kick plates where building supplies are sold.

126 Eliminate extra steps to open or unlock your exterior door by keeping an extra garage-door opener in the house. When you want to let someone into your locked house, press the battery-operated garage-door opener. The door to the garage will open and your guests can use the garage entrance to your house.

127   If arthritis affects your finger function, grasping and turning keys may be difficult. Enlarged key holders are available at some hardware stores. Ask your doctor or therapist about devices that are available to make keys easier to use.

INSTALLING POWER SWITCHES, ELECTRICAL CORDS AND SMALL APPLIANCES

128   When installing a light switch, always place it so you can illuminate a dark area before entering. This will help prevent falls that may cause trauma to already painful joints. Make light switches easier to see by using switch plates that are painted a color that contrasts with the wall paint, or by installing lighted switches (available from lighting-supply and discount stores).

129   Consider replacing traditional light switches with rocker-panel light switches that require less fine-motor control. These switches can be turned on by pressing with an arm, an elbow or the palm of the hand, and come lighted or unlighted. Find them at discount, building-supply or hardware stores.

130   A dimmer switch allows you to adjust the light in the room so that one person can work or read without disturbing others.

131 If electrical wall outlets are difficult to reach, you can use multiple-outlet power strips in every room of the house. The strips are inexpensive and plug right in to any household outlet. Place the strips where they are convenient to reach, and plug in appliances anywhere on the strip. These are safer than extension cords because most models have a circuit breaker or surge protector to prevent overloading. The strips are available at most discount and hardware stores.

132 Plug all your computer equipment into one power-strip surge protector so you can press one switch to turn on all the equipment at once.

133 Lamps are easier to turn on and off if you install a lamp converter. The converter bypasses the on-off switch and makes the entire lamp "touch sensitive." To install a converter, remove the light bulb and insert the converter into the socket. Then screw in a three-way light bulb. Touch the metal part of the lamp and a dim light will come on. Touch again and the light will get a little brighter. Touch a third time and the light will be its brightest. Touch again and the light goes off. These are available from many lighting and discount department stores.

134 Make sure that no loose electrical cords are left where you or members of your family might trip over them. Cord shorteners, which are reels that hold excess lamp-size cord, are available at lighting and discount department stores.

135 If it's difficult to dial a standard telephone, use a pencil or similar object to dial and reduce stress to your fingers. Or consider purchasing a large keypad telephone and use the palm of your hand to press the buttons. You can purchase this type of phone from your local telephone company or discount store.

136 Consider purchasing phones with an automatic dial feature. These phones dial your most frequently called numbers with the touch of just one button. Or contact your telephone company; many offer a speed-dialing service for a nominal fee.

137 A speaker phone makes using the telephone easier. You don't have to hold the receiver, and you can talk on the phone from up to 15 feet away. Speaker phones are available wherever traditional phones are sold.

IMPROVING FAUCETS AND SINKS

138 Turning water on and off is easier if you have a single lever arm to control the temperature and the amount of water coming out of the spout. Kitchen faucets usually have longer levers, so they are easier to use in both the kitchen and the bathroom. If you already own a bathroom faucet with a single lever arm, you may be able to replace the shorter lever with a kitchen-length lever.

139 If you have separate controls for hot and cold water, consider installing wrist blades. Wrist blades are wide, wing-type handles that can be operated by pushing with the forearm, wrist or heel of the hand. These are available at most plumbing suppliers or local hardware stores.

140 Automatic faucets are even easier to use. A sensor turns on the water when you put your hands under the faucet and stops the flow automatically when your hands are withdrawn. The water temperature can be set to a predetermined temperature. It's also possible to bypass the automatic feature and use it as a regular faucet. Contact a plumbing-supply store for more information and for installation advice.

ADAPTING FURNITURE, RUGS, WALLS AND STAIRS

141 Chairs and couches should be approximately 17 inches or higher off the ground so they're easier to get into or out of. Adjust the height of your furniture by adding or removing casters, adding seat cushions, or placing measured blocks of wood under each leg until the desired height is achieved.

142 If you need quiet time to rest and you're looking for ways to "soundproof" your house, here are some things you can do: Cover hardwood floors with carpet or area rugs; put up heavy, lined drapes; and, wherever possible, place upholstered furniture against the walls between rooms. You can also have hollow doors replaced with solid doors.

143 To help protect walls from being bumped and gouged by wheelchairs or scooters, put up sheets of clear plastic approximately ¼-inch thick at strategic locations.

144 If arthritis affects your hips or knees, going up and down the stairs can be taxing and painful. When climbing stairs, lead with your strong leg going up and your weak leg going down. Some people with arthritis find it helpful to walk at a sideways angle so they can hold the railing with both hands.

145 Stairways are a prime location for accidents. Here are a few tips to make stairs in your home as safe as possible: To prevent your feet from slipping on steps, consider adding abrasive rubber treads to carpeted stairs or clear or colored abrasive stair tape to uncarpeted stairs. Both products are available from hardware stores. To make basement stairs more visible, apply luminous paint to the edge of each step. For added safety, alternate between two colors of paint to keep from "missing" a step when you descend the stairs. Finally, be sure stairways are well lit. Whenever possible, have someone install sturdy railings, anchored to wall studs, on both sides of the stairs.

Remove small area rugs from your floors, especially in the kitchen. This is a prime location for slips and falls.

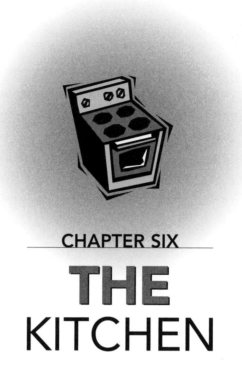

CHAPTER SIX

THE
KITCHEN

If your home is like most, the kitchen is probably the busiest room in your house. It's also the room where your body does more work than you may realize: stirring foods, grasping utensils, reaching high or low into cabinets, pulling drawers, lifting heavy pans or groceries. With a few minor adjustments and a little creativity, you can still accomplish these tasks while at the same time protecting your joints and conserving your energy.

The first step in kitchen planning is to arrange your kitchen for maximum efficiency. A conveniently planned kitchen does not have to be large or expensive. It must, however, be tailored to your needs. Creative rearranging can often save you money. For example, a cutting board placed over an open drawer gives you a lowered work surface. Have someone cut a hole in the board and you have a bowl holder. Suggestions on redesigning kitchens are available in family and home magazines as well as from your occupational therapist.

In this chapter, you'll learn simple ways to organize your kitchen so it is more efficient for you and your family. And you'll learn meal-planning and preparation techniques even Martha Stewart would appreciate.

PLANNING YOUR MEALS

147 Impulsive eating equals poor nutrition, while good meal planning leads to better nutrition. Try planning meals one week at a time and preparing your grocery list at the same time. You'll eat better, save money and make fewer midweek trips to the grocery store.

148 If you have difficulty planning meals, find a nutritionist or occupational therapist who understands your eating patterns and can suggest appropriate meal plans.

149 Post your weekly menu near the refrigerator. Vary your menu with one-dish meals that streamline preparation. Recipes for cooking a variety of one-dish meals are often featured in family and home magazines. For convenience, note recipe and cookbook pages on your weekly menu.

150 When planning meals, take advantage of the times you feel best to prepare ahead and freeze any parts of meals you can. You might make double recipes each night when you make dinner and freeze the leftovers so you'll have ready-made meals on days when you have a flare, your joints are particularly sore or your energy level is low.

151 Get family members involved in meal planning. Allow each member, including children, to plan meals and make or dictate a list of the ingredients needed.

SELECTING AND ORGANIZING SUPPLIES

152 Save time and energy in the kitchen by storing items near the places in which they are used. Keep one set of measuring cups and spoons with the silverware and another near the stove. Keep coffee mugs near the coffee pot. Keep a measuring cup inside your flour or sugar canisters. Store microwave supplies including microwave-safe containers, plastic wrap and dye-free paper towels in one cupboard in the kitchen.

153 Spices are easier to find and use if you store them in alphabetical order in a kitchen drawer instead of a high cupboard.

154 Remove the magnetic door catches on difficult-to-open cabinet doors. Install hardware on the outside of cabinets that is easy to grasp. If doors are too hard to use, remove them and hang fabric curtains.

155 Good lighting reduces fatigue and the risk of accidents. Have someone install under-cabinet lights in your kitchen workspaces. The lights come in a variety of sizes and styles and are available from hardware and lighting-supply stores.

156 Add storage space by installing hooks under kitchen cabinets. Create a space for pots and pans by installing a pegboard or cast-iron wall fixture. Hang small gadgets and pot holders on the side of the refrigerator using magnetic hooks.

157 Store baking pans and trays in a cupboard that is equipped with vertical dividers. The pans can stand up between dividers, eliminating the need to lift several to get to the one on the bottom. Check with a carpenter or kitchen-cabinet supplier about installing the dividers.

158 Use separate wastebaskets for recyclables and trash. Help family members remember which is which by keeping recyclables on the right or by labeling the containers. Delegate the task of emptying these containers to another family member. See also Tip #117.

159 Store flour, sugar and coffee in plastic containers with handles and easy-to-remove lids, rather than in hard-to-use metal canisters. Keep them on the counter to avoid having to reach for and lift heavy containers.

160 Keep a small flashlight in the kitchen to make it easier to find items in the back of deep cupboards.

161 If it's difficult to lift and hold objects, consider replacing heavy dishes and cookware. Purchase lightweight dinner dishes — they're easier to lift and carry. Replace heavy pottery mugs with porcelain, china or insulated drinking cups. Use aluminum cookware, gadgets with big cushioned handles, sharp knives and lightweight stainless steel bowls to help you conserve strength and energy.

162 Use knives designed to lessen the strain on your hands by allowing you to use your entire arm when cutting foods. An ergonomically designed knife has a large handle almost perpendicular to the blade. The handle allows you to "saw" back and forth when cutting.

A rocker knife has a curved blade that you rock back and forth to cut food. Contact hospital rehabilitation centers or your local home-health stores to locate these types of knives.

163 Use a pastry blender to mix foods. Its large, thick handle makes it easier to use than a fork or mixing spoon.

USING YOUR KITCHEN APPLIANCES
AND EQUIPMENT

164 A stove with switches on the front rather than the back makes cooking easier for people with limited reaching abilities and for those seated in a wheelchair.

165 If you have difficulty turning the knobs on your stove or oven, you can adapt them by purchasing a universal turning aid that you attach to the knob. Ask your therapist for information on where to purchase this helpful device.

166 The refrigerator door will close automatically if you raise the front by placing a thin object under the front bottom edge.

167 If opening the refrigerator door is difficult, try tying a loop of fabric or cord around the handle. Use the loop to pull the door open with your forearm to avoid putting unnecessary strain on your hands and joints.

The door is also easier to open if you place one or two strips of electrical tape across the bottom gasket. The appliance may be less energy efficient, but you'll need less strength to open the door.

168 If you ever have a need to purée food, purchase a blender that accommodates small, individual blender jars you can purchase separately. Then blend each food in a separate container. You'll retain the individual taste of the foods you purée.

169   Use an electric frying pan or wok so you can sit at the kitchen table while you cook.

PREPARING YOUR MEALS

170   Peeled and cut vegetables like carrots and celery are an easy, make-ahead snack. Keep them fresh and crisp by putting them in a zipper-type bag with an ice cube or two, and store in the refrigerator. Many grocery stores sell cut vegetables in their produce section, and some may even cut or chop your produce upon request.

171   When baking, place baking dishes and pie pans on a baking sheet, shallow roasting pan or jelly-roll pan lined with aluminum foil. The dishes will be easier to lift, and the larger outer pans will catch spill-overs.

172   If you're cooking and cleaning up from a wheelchair, purchase or make a towel that drapes over the arm of your wheelchair and fastens with a button to keep it from falling off. The towel comes in handy for all kinds of purposes.

173   If you need to sit while cooking, have an adjustable mirror mounted over the stove. Angle the mirror so you can more easily see into the pots and pans while you cook.

174 When cooking from a wheelchair or while sitting down, create a lowered work space by setting a plastic cutting board or cookie sheet over an open drawer. Be sure the drawer has a safety catch to prevent it from sliding completely out of its slot. See Tip #38.

175 Use disposable plastic gloves to protect your hands from the cold while mixing meat loaf, making hamburger patties or handling other cold foods. If you have Raynaud's phenomenon, further protect your fingers from the cold by wearing insulated gloves underneath.

176 At holiday time, try baking with friends in assembly-line fashion. Have everyone bring a favorite recipe and necessary ingredients. You can choose a job that's easier on your joints or one that can be done sitting down.

177 Keep recipe cards handy while in use by inserting them between the tines of a fork, then placing the fork in a glass. The cards stay clean and easy to read.

178 If bending is hard on your back, keep a small wastebasket on the counter during meal preparation. Line the basket with a recycled plastic bag and toss in vegetable peels, empty packages, cans, etc. When you're finished cooking, discard everything at once in the kitchen wastebasket.

179 Attach small casters or wheels to the underside of a cutting board. Use the adapted cutting board as a trivet or to move heavy pots or dishes from one place to another.

180 It's easier to drain cooked spaghetti if you put a colander with cool-to-the-touch handles inside the cooking pan and then add the pasta. When the spaghetti is cooked, simply lift out the colander. Purchase a handled colander wherever better cookware is sold.

181 Broiler pans are easier to clean if you pour a cup of water into the bottom portion of the pan before cooking. The water keeps drippings from being baked on and eliminates smoke during cooking.

182 Some foods are easier to handle or prepare when frozen. Cutting or slicing meat, fish or chicken is easier when it's frozen slightly. For sandwich preparation, peanut butter, jelly, margarine and other fillings spread easier if the bread is frozen. The bread doesn't tear, and it defrosts so quickly that by the time you finish the task and get to the table, the sandwich is ready to eat. It's also easier to frost and slice a cake that's been frozen. The cake will thaw as you frost and slice it.

183 Whenever possible, select whipped butter and cream cheese. These products are much easier to spread than the other varieties of butter and cheese.

184 If you have trouble separating eggs, use a small aluminum kitchen funnel. Place the funnel in a measuring cup and break the egg into it. The white slips neatly and easily into the cup, and the yolk stays in the funnel.

185 Always crack eggs on the rim of an empty bowl. If pieces of the shell fall into the bowl, they'll be easier to remove. The thinner the rim of the bowl, the easier it is to get a clean crack. If this method is too difficult, hold the egg about 10 or 12 inches above an empty bowl and drop it into the bowl. The egg will break in two, making the shell easy to remove, even for those with limited fine-motor control.

186 Beating eggs is easier if you use a wire whisk or electric blender. Another easy alternative is to break the eggs into a jar, replace the lid and shake the jar.

187 To peel hard-cooked eggs, drain the water from the pot and shake the pot vigorously. Then run the eggs under cold water. The shells will slip off easily.

188 Boil potatoes and other vegetables in a metal frying basket or cool-handle colander that has been set inside a larger pot. When the potatoes are done, lift out the basket or colander. Let the pot of hot water cool before you transfer it to the sink.

189 Open the pull-top tab on a can of soda by lifting the tab just high enough to hook it into a cup hook that you've screwed onto the underside of a kitchen cabinet. Once the tab is hooked, pull gently and the tab will pop up. Alternatively, if you have the hand strength, try using a staple remover to grasp and lift up the tab.

190 Freeze leftovers as complete dinners. Put serving-size portions of leftover food on a microwave-safe plate and cover it first with plastic wrap, then with aluminum foil. The double wraps will protect the food from freezer burn. When you're ready to use it, remove the foil, make a small cut in the plastic wrap, and warm the meal in the microwave.

191 If you don't have a microwave or toaster oven, you can conserve energy and save on clean-up time when you heat small amounts of leftovers wrapped in individual aluminum foil packages. Place the packages side by side in a frying pan containing an inch of water and heat over a single burner. This way there is only one pan to wash.

192 If traditional cookie cutters are hard to use, try using a metal, glass or hard-plastic tumbler. Dip the tumbler in flour or use vegetable cooking spray before each use so the dough won't stick.

193 To close bread bags without a twist tie, hold the open end of the bag and twist it around several times. Then, open the bag just above the twisted neck and pull it back over the loaf of bread.

194 Instead of shaking bottles and jars, roll them on a counter top or table. To make opening the jar easier, refer to Tip #49. If scraping down the sides of almost-empty jars of jelly, mayonnaise, mustard, relish, etc., is a problem, store them on their sides.

195 Cover your hand with a clear plastic sandwich bag before you grease baking pans. This way, you can use your entire hand to grease your baking pan if you'd like, without getting grease on your hands.

196 If you bake a cake in a spring-form pan, you can remove it with one hand.

SETTING AND CLEARING THE TABLE

197 Drinking glasses with bumpy exteriors are easier to grasp than glasses with smooth exteriors. If you only have smooth drinking glasses, make them easier to grasp by having someone wind two rubber bands tightly around the glass about an inch or so apart. Also look for smaller, light-weight varieties.

198 Cups with handles and thumb rests on each side make handling beverages easier. Look for these special cups at home-health stores or in mail-order catalogs.

199 Purchase plates with a high outer edge. They keep food from sliding off the plate while you're eating.

200 Cutting your food is easier if you use a rubber suction soap holder to secure a plate to the table.

201 To save time setting the table, wrap individual place settings of silverware in napkins. Keep the wrapped silverware in a basket near the table.

202 Getting a wheelchair close enough to the dinner table to comfortably eat a meal can be difficult. The armrests are often too high to fit under the table. Here's a solution for creating your new custom place mat. Place a jelly-roll pan (a cookie sheet with sides) or a cafeteria tray lengthwise across the armrests. If these aren't wide enough to rest across the armrests of your wheelchair, then have someone cut a board that is the appropriate dimensions for your needs. Then push the wheelchair close to the table and allow the edge of your tray to rest flush with the edge of the table. Put your plate and drink on your new custom place mat.

203 If it's difficult to extend your arm to reach your plate, try elevating your plate. Experiment with different heights. Use a wicker bread basket, a book or a sturdy cardboard box to raise the plate to the appropriate height.

204 Use a mixture of water and household ammonia to remove baked-on foods. Pour one-half cup of ammonia into the pan, add water, stir and cover tightly. The next day, the baked-on foods will virtually slide off the pan. Be careful to rinse the pan thoroughly before using any cleaning products that contain chlorine bleach; mixing the two chemicals creates toxic fumes.

205 If you have a weak grasp or drop things frequently when washing dishes, try washing them in a plastic tub that is placed inside the sink. Alternatively, you could line the bottom of the sink with a rubber mat, towel or sponge-type mat.

206 When washing dishes, place an upside down plastic dish drainer or utility basket in the sink. Dishes will sit on top of it so they're easier to reach. When scrubbing, try using large sponges or handled scrubbers to make washing easier. If possible, keep your fingers extended in order to reduce stress on your joints.

207 Make kitchen clean-up easier for everyone. Require each family member to clear and wash his or her own dishes. Establish the rule that no one leaves the kitchen until it is clean.

CREATING A SAFE KITCHEN

208 Use pans on burners that are approximately the same size as the bottom of the pan. Turn handles inward to avoid knocking pots and pans off the stove.

209 Hot dishes are safer to handle using oven mitts instead of hot pads.

210 Lift lids off pots and pans slowly, tipping the lid so the steam escapes away from you. Wearing long, tapered sleeves keeps steam from burning your arms when cooking.

211 If conventional step stools are difficult to move from one location to another, consider purchasing a stool with self-locking wheels, like those found in libraries. The stools are available at office-supply stores and push easily over vinyl flooring or kitchen carpet.

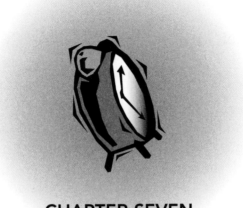

CHAPTER SEVEN

THE
BEDROOM

If you have arthritis, you are accustomed to the fatigue that may accompany joint and muscle pain. When your arthritis is particularly active, it is often helpful to take longer and more frequent rest breaks. Maintaining the correct position in bed for your type of arthritis is important. Your bed, mattress pad, sheets, pillows and blankets also determine how comfortably you rest.

In this chapter, you'll learn ways to create a bedroom that's warm and inviting. You'll also learn not only how to set up and organize your bedroom, but how to be more comfortable in bed when you want to catch a few winks.

SELECTING FURNITURE AND ACCESSORIES

212 A good bed is firm enough to support your body while you are lying in the position that's best for you, and it distributes pressure evenly. Use a firm mattress or add extra support by placing a $1/2$-inch-thick plywood board or bedboard underneath the mattress.

213 You'll be more comfortable in bed if you choose the right bedding and equipment for your needs. Always look for bed covers that provide warmth without weight. Woven knit sheets are easy to put on the mattress because the corners stretch easily, but if turning over in bed is difficult, woven satin sheets will help you slide more easily (especially if you wear nylon tricot pajamas).

214 If you need to avoid excessive pressure from bedding on your feet and toes, try making a simple footboard from a piece of wood, or use a cardboard box. Place the wooden board or box at the end of the bed and drape the covers over it. The covers will lay across the footboard without touching your feet and toes.

215 It's easier to get out of bed if the bed is about the same height as your knees when you are standing. If you have knee problems, the bed should be higher so you can easily get into and out of the bed. If the bed is too tall, have a carpenter cut the legs. If it's too low, use a thicker mattress or try adding a mattress pad. Or, have someone elevate the bed by placing the legs on blocks.

216 Mattress life can be extended by having the mattress turned periodically (both end to end and top to bottom). Keep track of how and when the mattress was rotated by keeping a dated index card between the mattress and box spring. The mattress will not only last longer, it will better support your back to help prevent back pain.

217 For comfort and convenience, a cabinet beside the bed can be used to hold a telephone and important phone numbers, water, reading material, correspondence and medications. If you have younger visitors, you could keep crayons and books nearby, but be sure medications are out of sight and in childproof containers. If you have trouble opening childproof containers, store your medications in a lock box that children cannot get into.

218 In a pinch, an adjustable ironing board makes a good nightstand or bedside table. It holds a number of items and can be adjusted to the right height.

219 Keep a flashlight near the entrance to the bedroom. Use it at night when you've turned off the light and need to see to get to bed. The flashlight also comes in handy if you have to get out of bed in the middle of the night.

220   If you need the bedroom to be absolutely dark in order to sleep, purchase room-darkening shades. These inexpensive shades can be cut to fit almost any window and can be found wherever drapes and curtains are sold.

MAKING YOUR BEDROOM MORE ACCESSIBLE AND COMFORTABLE

221   To get bed sheets and blankets to hang evenly on both sides, mark the center of the top sheet and blanket in some way, perhaps by using an indelible marker or ironing on a decorative decal. Then put the marker in the middle of the bed, and the bed covering will be centered.

222   Make it easier to sit up or get out of bed by pushing the side of the bed against a bedroom wall and installing a railing or grab bar. Lie in bed to see where and how high the railing or bar should be installed. Grab bars or railings should always be anchored to a stud in the wall.

223   If you or someone in your family must spend extended periods of time in bed, try to position the bed so that he or she can see out a window or door. The change of scenery helps ease boredom and feelings of isolation.

224 If it's difficult to roll over in bed, try making a simple loop chain. Purchase flexible, strong belt material. Have someone sew the material into 10-inch loops, then sew the loops together to form a chain. Install the chain on the far side of the bed, attaching it either to a bed rail that slips between the mattress and box spring or, if your mattress is so equipped, to the handles that are used to help turn the mattress. You can grasp the chain to help pull yourself into a new position.

225 A trapeze-type device attached to the bedboard or installed in the ceiling above the bed also makes sitting up and changing positions easier. Contact an occupational therapist or ask your physician for advice on what to purchase or how to make such a device.

226 Make it easy to keep bedrooms looking nice by replacing heavy bedspreads with an attractive top sheet, blanket or sleeping bag. Add a dust ruffle for a finished look. The bed will be easier to make, and the bedding will be easier to launder.

227 If you use a top sheet and blanket, try pinning them together so you can pull them up at the same time when making the bed. Have someone sew loops to the top of the covers so that you can pull them up with your arms.

228 In case of an emergency, it's a good idea to keep a flash-light, some matches and a candle by the bedside. Keep a pair of shoes by the bed to protect your feet in case there's any broken glass.

229 Use a plastic cup with a lid that holds a flexible straw (often called a sports bottle) for drinking water during the night. If you accidentally knock the water over, only a few drops will spill before you set the cup upright. The flexible straw makes it easier to drink beverages if you must drink while reclining.

230 If you are confined to bed, you can increase your reachable space by putting a turntable on the nightstand. Also, keep a reacher nearby so you can retrieve items that drop on the floor without getting out of bed. For information on reach-ers, see Tips #37 and #51.

231 If you use an electric blanket to provide warmth, try turning on the heat for 20 minutes before getting up to reduce stiff-ness in your joints. Fleece or electric mattress pads provide additional warmth from below the body. Down duvets are lightweight covers but still provide adequate warmth.

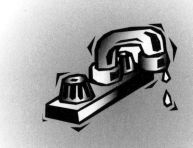

CHAPTER EIGHT

THE BATHROOM

No doubt taking care of our personal needs independently is important to all of us. The bathroom is not only the most important location for these tasks, but it is also the site of frequent accidents. In this chapter, you'll learn about simple techniques and devices that can make many personal-care tasks easier. And the bathrooms in your home will be more accessible, safer and easier for you to use.

ORGANIZING THE BATHROOM

232 Keep a teaspoon or measuring spoon in one of the slots of your toothbrush holder so that you have a spoon handy in the bathroom for taking medicine. Or hang a set of measuring spoons from an adhesive-backed hook inside the door of the medicine cabinet.

233 If counter space is limited, hang a ceramic pot in a macrame plant hanger from the ceiling in the bathroom. Use it to hold daily-use items such as toothpaste, cotton balls, deodorant, etc.

MAKING YOUR BATHROOM SAFER AND MORE ACCESSIBLE

234 If moving in and out of the bathtub or shower is difficult, have safety rails or grab bars installed. Do not use a towel bar or soap dish holder to lean on. These are not strong enough to support your body weight. Ask your therapist for advice on what type of safety rails to purchase.

235 If you or someone in your home temporarily uses a wheelchair, you can make it easier to access the bathroom by replacing the door with an opaque shower curtain hung on cafe rings from a tension rod. It's an inexpensive way to address a temporary problem.

236 If your reaching or bending capabilities are limited, use long-handled bath sponges or brushes to make bathing easier.

237 Bath chairs or benches that you place in the tub or shower stall allow you to sit while you shower. Check your local pharmacy or home-health supply store for selection and prices.

238 A raised toilet seat may make it easier for you to lower yourself to the toilet, since you do not have to go down as far to use the seat. It also helps you to stand up again. If you use your hands to assist in moving onto and off of the toilet seat, be sure to open your fingers and use the palm of your hands for pushing. Raised toilet seats are available at your local pharmacy or home-health supply store.

239 Rubber mats in the bathtub help reduce the risk of slipping and falling; however, with use, a soapy film can collect on the surface, eventually making the mat just as slippery as the tub surface. If you periodically wash the mat in the washing machine with some soap and a little bleach, it will be as good as new.

240 Try using soap-on-a-rope or liquid soap in a pump dispenser to keep soap from slipping from your hands when you are showering or bathing.

241 It's easier to get out of the tub safely if you wring out a washcloth and use it to help grasp the edge of the tub. Use lightweight cotton dishcloths instead of terrycloth wash-cloths — they're easier to wring out. If arthritis makes wringing out a washcloth difficult, purchase a wash mitt that you can press with a flat hand.

242 The bathtub or shower is a good place to do range-of-motion or isometric exercises and arm exercises. The warmth and buoyancy of the water may ease motion and make exercising less painful. Ask your physician or therapist for more information about these and other exercises.

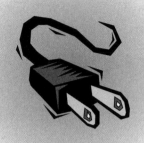

CHAPTER NINE

HOUSEHOLD
SAFETY

Do you know where the fuse box is in your house? Do you have the proper number of smoke detectors in your home? Creating a safe environment in your home is a major responsibility, and it's easier if you plan ahead. If you have arthritis or know someone else living with a chronic condition, you'll benefit greatly from the no-nonsense tips for a safer household available in this chapter. In addition, local safety councils have pamphlets available to assist you in thoroughly assessing the safety of your home.

243 Those who use power-dependent life-support equipment, like oxygen, hemodialysis or sleep apnea machines, should advise their electric companies of their use before an emergency power outage occurs. Your doctor will be asked to fill out a form indicating your medical problem and the type of equipment you use. In an emergency, the utility company will make every attempt to restore service as soon as possible, but it is still the customer's responsibility to have a backup power source.

244 Electric beds, lifts and environmental-control units are also considered life-support equipment. If you use any of these, the electric company will tag your meter. When repairs, meter changes or routine maintenance necessitate that power be suspended, customers with tagged meters will be notified ahead of time so they can make arrangements. Check with your electric company about having this done.

245 Notify your local fire department if you think you would have difficulty escaping from your home in the event of a fire. If a fire is reported, the dispatcher will tell fire fighters where in the building to look for persons needing assistance, and whether special equipment or rescue procedures might be necessary. In some communities, information is not shared by the fire, police and other emergency medical services, so you may need to contact each agency independently.

246 Keep fire extinguishers in various places throughout your home where fires might occur, especially in the kitchen and workshop areas. When selecting a fire extinguisher, make sure that you understand how to use the controls and be certain that you are able to lift and activate the extinguisher.

247 Although most people have at least one smoke alarm somewhere in the house, it's important to have alarms in several locations, including all sleeping areas, the basement and the kitchen. Carbon monoxide detectors are just as important as smoke detectors. Refer to the manufacturer's instructions to determine how many you need and where they should be installed.

248 If young children will be visiting, be sure to take simple childproofing measures. Fold tablecloths and table runners up onto the table rather than letting them hang over the side where they could be pulled down along with whatever is on the table. Put medicines, cleaning supplies and other poisonous household substances out of reach. For extended visits, consider adding a temporary handrail at child height on the wall opposite the permanent handrail on frequently used stairways; install a safety gate at the top or bottom of stairs to keep toddlers from using the stairs. Remember, all grab bars and railings should be anchored to a stud in the wall.

249

Show all family members where the main water shut-off valve is located and teach them how and when to use it. To keep the valve in good working order, turn it off and on every six months.

250

Be sure all family members know where the fuse box or circuit breaker is located and how to turn off the electricity in your house. In addition, label each switch in the circuit breaker or fuse box so you know at a glance which circuit serves each room and each appliance.

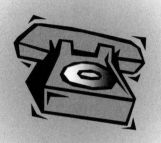

RESOURCES

ABOUT THE ARTHRITIS FOUNDATION

The Arthritis Foundation is the source of help and hope for nearly 40 million Americans who have arthritis. Founded in 1948, the Arthritis Foundation is the only national, voluntary health organization that works for all people affected by any of the more than 100 forms of arthritis or related diseases. Volunteers in chapters nationwide help to support research, professional and community education programs, services for people with arthritis, government advocacy and fund-raising activities.

The American Juvenile Arthritis Organization (AJAO) is composed of children, parents, teachers and others who are concerned specifically about juvenile arthritis. A council of the

Arthritis Foundation, AJAO focuses its efforts on the problems related to arthritis in children.

The focus of the Arthritis Foundation is two-fold: to support research to find the cure for and prevention of arthritis, and to improve the quality of life for those affected by arthritis. Public contributions enable the Arthritis Foundation to fulfill this mission — in fact, at least 80 cents of every dollar donated to the Arthritis Foundation serves to directly fund research, programs and services.

THE ARTHRITIS FOUNDATION HELPS

Arthritis doesn't have to rob you of the activities you enjoy most. While research holds the key to future cures for and prevention of arthritis, the Arthritis Foundation believes it is equally important to improve the quality of life for people with arthritis today. The chapter that serves your area has information, classes and other services to put you in charge of your arthritis. The Arthritis Foundation has more than 150 offices across the United States. To find the office near you, call 800/283-7800. Contact the chapter in your area to find out which of the following resources it has available.

MEDICAL AND SELF-CARE PROGRAMS

1. **Physician referral** — Most Arthritis Foundation chapters can provide a list of doctors in your area who specialize in the evaluation and treatment of arthritis and arthritis-related diseases.

2. **Exercise programs** — Recreational in nature, these are developed, coordinated and sponsored by the Arthritis Foundation. All have specially trained instructors. They include:

   - **Joint Efforts** — This arthritis movement program teaches gentle, undemanding movement exercises for people with arthritis, including those who use walkers and wheelchairs. Joint Efforts is designed to encourage movement and socialization among older adults and to help decrease pain, stiffness and depression.
   - **PACE® (People with Arthritis Can Exercise)** — PACE® is an exercise program that uses gentle activities to help increase joint flexibility, range of motion and stamina, and to help maintain muscle strength. Two videotapes showing basic and advanced levels of the program are available from your chapter for preview or for practice at home. To purchase the videos, call 800/933-0032.
   - **Arthritis Foundation Aquatic Program** — Originally co-developed by the YMCA and the Arthritis Foundation, this water-exercise program helps relieve the strain on muscles and joints for people with arthritis.

The PEP (Pool Exercise Program) videotape shows how to exercise on your own. To order the video, call 800/933-0032.

EDUCATIONAL AND
EMOTIONAL SUPPORT GROUPS

1. **Arthritis Foundation Support and Education Groups —** These are mutual-support groups that provide opportunities for discussion and problem solving. They are usually formed by people with arthritis and/or their family members who wish to meet with their peers for mutual assistance in satisfying common needs and in overcoming problems related to arthritis.

2. **Classes/courses —** In these formal group meetings, people with various types of arthritis can gain the knowledge, skills and confidence they need to actively manage their conditions. Courses focus on proper exercises, medications, relaxation techniques, pain management, dealing with depression, nutrition, nontraditional treatments and doctor-patient relations. The classes include:
   - **Arthritis Self-Help Course**
   - **Fibromyalgia Self-Help Course**
   - **Systemic Lupus Erythematosus Self-Help Course**

RELIABLE INFORMATION AT YOUR FINGERTIPS

1. **Information hotline** — The Arthritis Foundation is the authority on arthritis and is only a phone call away. Call toll free at 800/283-7800 for automated information on arthritis 24 hours a day. Trained volunteers and staff are also available at your local Arthritis Foundation to answer your questions or send you a list of physicians in your area who specialize in arthritis.

2. **Arthritis Foundation website** — Information about arthritis is available 24 hours a day to Internet users via the Arthritis Foundation's site on the World Wide Web. The address for the website is http://www.arthritis.org.

3. **Publications** — A number of publications are available to educate people with arthritis and their families and friends about important considerations such as medications, exercise, diet, pain management and stress management, to name a few.

- **Booklets** — More than 60 booklets and brochures provide information on the many arthritis-related diseases and conditions, medications, guidance for working with your doctor and caring for yourself. Single copies are available free of charge. Call 800/283-7800 for a free listing of booklets on arthritis.

- *Arthritis Today* — The award-winning bimonthly magazine, *Arthritis Today,* gives you the latest information on research, new treatments and tips from experts and readers to help you manage arthritis. Each issue also brings you a variety of helpful and interesting articles covering diet and nutrition, tips for traveling and ways you can make your life with arthritis easier and more rewarding. A one-year subscription to *Arthritis Today* is yours free when you become a member of the Arthritis Foundation. Annual membership is $20 and helps fund research to find cures for arthritis. Call 800/933-0032 for membership and subscription information.

- **Books** — Self-help books are available from the Arthritis Foundation to help you learn more about your condition and how to manage it. Check your local bookstores, your local Arthritis Foundation chapter, or order a book through the Arthritis Foundation by calling 800/207-8633.

4. **Audiovisual libraries** — Available either on loan or for purchase, audio- and videocassettes cover a variety of topics from exercise to relaxation. Call the chapter that serves your area for a listing of titles, prices and availability.

5. **Speakers' bureaus** — Lay and professional volunteers conduct educational presentations to different groups. To schedule a speaker for your group, call the chapter that serves your area.

6. **Public forums** — Educational programs are presented to the community on various requested topics.

7. **Professional publications** — A number of professional educational materials on arthritis geared to the health-care professional are available through the Arthritis Foundation. These materials include the *Bulletin on the Rheumatic Diseases,* a newsletter published eight times a year. For subscription information, call 404/872-7100. The 356-page *Primer on the Rheumatic Diseases,* published every five years, is available by calling 800/207-8633.

REMEMBER THE ARTHRITIS FOUNDATION IN YOUR WILL

Planned giving is an important part of fulfilling the Arthritis Foundation's mission to support arthritis research and improve the quality of life for those affected by arthritis. The Arthritis Foundation offers a wide variety of gift planning options — gifts of cash, appreciated assets, gifts by will or living trust, naming the Arthritis Foundation as beneficiary of your life insurance, individual retirement account (IRA), pension, 401(k) or other retirement savings plan.

It is our hope that you decide to include a gift to the Arthritis Foundation in your will. Your greatest benefit in assisting the Arthritis Foundation will be the personal satisfaction of making a difference in the struggle against arthritis. For more information on giving opportunities, call the planned giving department at 404/872-7100.

Arthritis Foundation
1330 W. Peachtree Street
Atlanta, GA 30309
404/872-7100
800/283-7800
http://www.arthritis.org